Keto Mediterranean Recipe

The Optimal Keto-Friendly Diet with Flavorful Low-Carb Mediterranean Recipes

Kendra Harrison

© Copyright 2021 by - Kendra Harrison - All rights reserved.

The following Book is reproduced below with the goal of providing information that is as accurate and reliable as possible. Regardless, purchasing this Book can be seen as consent to the fact that both the publisher and the author of this book are in no way experts on the topics discussed within and that any recommendations or suggestions that are made herein are for entertainment purposes only. Professionals should be consulted as needed prior to undertaking any of the action endorsed herein.

This declaration is deemed fair and valid by both the American Bar Association and the Committee of Publishers Association and is legally binding throughout the United States.

Furthermore, the transmission, duplication, or reproduction of any of the following work including specific information will be considered an illegal act irrespective of if it is done electronically or in print. This extends to creating a secondary or tertiary copy of the work or a recorded copy and is only allowed with the express written consent from the Publisher. All additional right reserved.

The information in the following pages is broadly considered a truthful and accurate account of facts and as such, any inattention, use, or misuse of the information in question by the reader will render any resulting actions solely under their purview. There are no scenarios in which the publisher or the original author of this work can be in any fashion deemed liable for any hardship or damages that may befall them after undertaking information described herein.

Additionally, the information in the following pages is intended only for informational purposes and should thus be thought of as universal. As befitting its nature, it is presented without assurance regarding its prolonged validity or interim quality. Trademarks that are mentioned are done without written consent and can in no way be considered an endorsement from the trademark holder.

Table of Contents

Introduction 7

Keto Mediterranean Recipes 9

    Oatmeal with Yogurt and Egg 10

    Tomato Eggs 11

    Low-Carb Keto Waffles 12

    Greek Bowl 13

    Scrambled Eggs, Med Style 14

    Warm Pumpkin Oats 15

    Caprese Breakfast Muffin 16

    Buffalo Chicken Chaffle 17

    Savory Egg Galettes 19

    Breakfast Cobbler 20

    Carrot Chaffle Cake 21

    Avocado Wrapped in Bacon 23

    Roasted Veggies 24

    Mini Keto Pizza 25

    Healthy Tuna Wraps 27

    Salmon with a Pesto Crust 29

    Keto Calamari 30

    Courgette Grilled Cheese 31

    Pork Loin with Cauliflower Mash 33

    Orange and Fennel Salad 35

    Guacamole with Coriander and Limes 36

Caponata Lamb	37
Grilled Shrimp Salad	39
Mediterranean Stuffed Tomatoes	41
Cheesy Spinach Chicken	42
Simple Tomato Soup	44
Chicken and Shrimp	45
Warming Fish Stew	47
Tuscan Chicken Skillet	48
Caprese Salad	50
Spanish Chilled Soup	51
Skinny Bruschetta Chicken	52
Easy Parmesan Crusted Tilapia	53
Crabmeat, Prosciutto, and Vegetable Delight	54
Fully Stuffed Peppers	55
Scallops Provencal	57
Roasted Lemon Asparagus	59
Sicilian Marinated Olives	60
Fig and Anise Ice Cream	61
Healthier Brownies	63
Honey Yogurt with Balsamic Berries	65
Ricotta Cake	66
Coco Macaroons	67
Caramel Cookies	68
Pecans with Caramel	69

Chocolate Cake 70

Vanilla Pears 71

Apple Pie 73

Pumpkin Pie Flan 75

Cheesecake Cupcakes 77

Introduction

The **Mediterranean Diet** focuses on healthy and delicious foods. If you have been struggling to adhere to a more healthy way of eating, want to be able to cut out the processed and pre-packaged foods from your diet, and want to stress less about your health, then the Mediterranean diet is your solution. This inexpensive diet is satisfying and easy to follow.

To many people, the best benefit of the Mediterranean diet is that you are able to lose weight by making healthier eating decisions. You do not have to starve yourself or reduce your food portions, but by naturally shifting to healthier foods, you can lose weight and keep that weight off. It depends on which foods you are eating to gain your nutrients.

The **Keto Diet** is a low-carb, high-fat diet. This diet ultimately helps you... burning fat! How is that possible? When you eat a lot of carbohydrates, such as pasta, your metabolism turns carbs into glucose for energy.

The metabolic state where you burn fat instead of carbs for fuel is called ketosis. In such a state, your body produces ketones, an alternative source of fuel.

A typical standard American diet is normally high in carbs and refined foods, so switching to a ketogenic lifestyle can be tough at first. This big collection of delicious, simple, and affordable recipes will help you make your meals enjoyable and, more importantly, make your diet sustainable in the long term.

Keto Mediterranean Diet Recipes is a mix of both of these two diets. You will taste the best Mediterranean food adapted to the Ketogenic Diet.

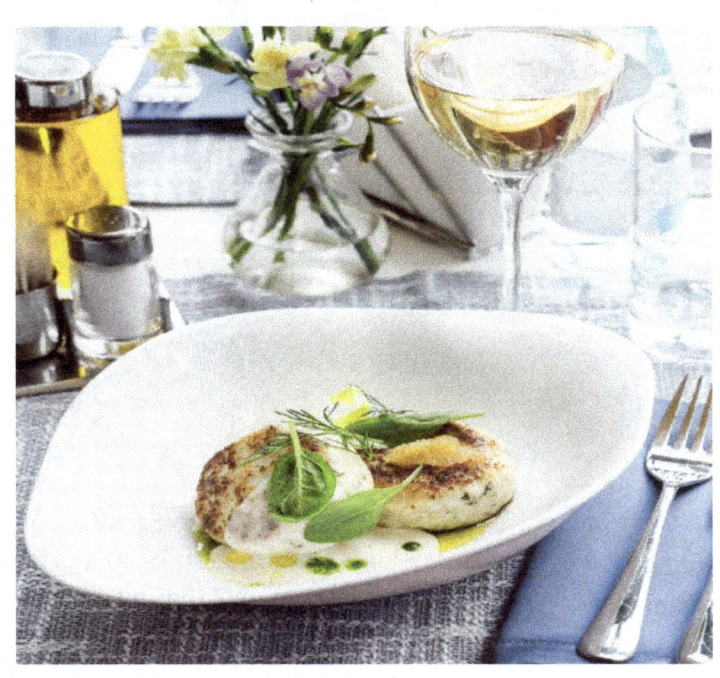

Keto Mediterranean Recipes

Oatmeal with Yogurt and Egg

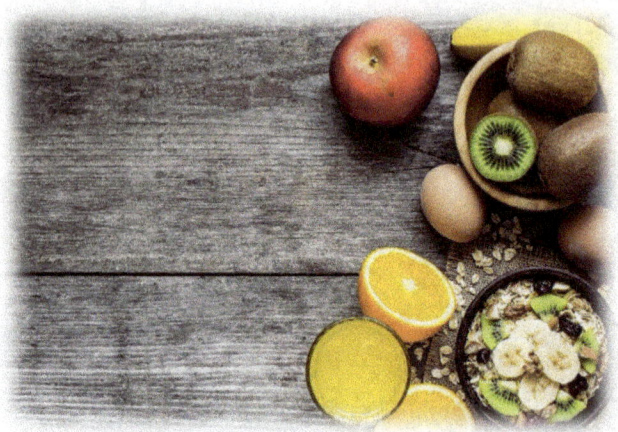

Time required: 7 minutes

Servings: 01

INGREDIENTS

⅓ c. oats
⅓ c. low-fat milk
1 egg
¼ tsp. cinnamon
¼ c. yogurt
¼ c. slashed apple
Salt
Sugar

STEPS FOR COOKING

1. Blend the milk and egg. Mix in all ingredients except yogurt and apple. Microwave until the liquid is evaporated, (for about 2 minutes).
2. Spread yogurt and apples on top of oatmeal.

Tomato Eggs

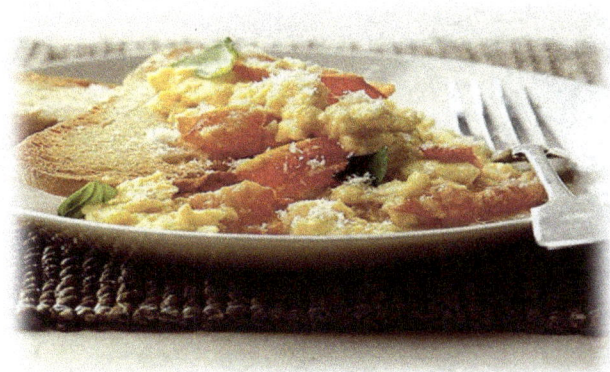

Time required: 10 minutes

Servings: 02

INGREDIENTS	STEPS FOR COOKING
1 tomato, chopped *1 teaspoon sunflower oil* *1 cup fresh parsley, chopped* *3 eggs, beaten* *1 oz. Feta cheese, crumbled*	1. Heat sunflower oil in the pan. 2. Then add chopped tomatoes and parsley. Cook the ingredients for 2 minutes. 3. After this, add eggs and stir the mixture well, then cook the dish for 2 minutes more. Add feta cheese and stir well. 4. Cook the meal for 1 more minute.

Low-Carb Keto Waffles

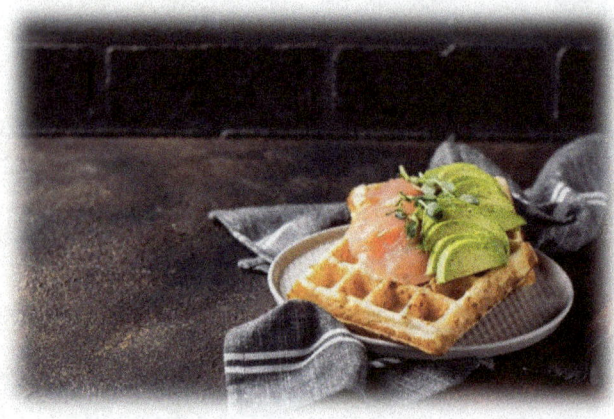

Time required: 20 minutes

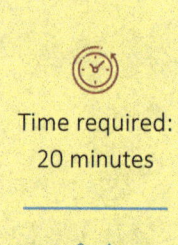

Servings: 02

INGREDIENTS

1 tablespoon of almond flour
1 egg
1 teaspoon vanilla
1 shake of cinnamon
1 teaspoon baking powder
1 cup mozzarella cheese

STEPS FOR COOKING

1. In a bowl, mix together, egg and vanilla extract.
2. Mix in baking powder, almond flour, and cinnamon.
3. Lastly, add in the mozzarella cheese and coat it evenly with the mixture.
4. Spray your waffle maker with oil and let it heat up to its highest setting.
5. Cook the waffle, checking on it every 5 minutes until it gets crunchy and golden. A tip: Make sure you put in half of your batter. The waffle maker can overflow, making it a messy process. I suggest putting down a silpat mat for an easy clean up.
6. Take it out carefully, and top it with butter, and your favorite low-carb syrup.

Greek Bowl

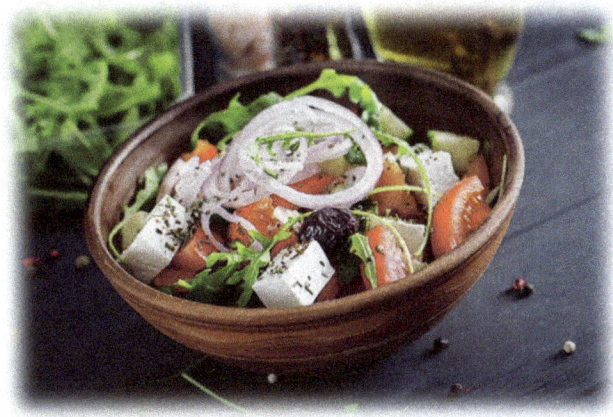

Time required: 17 minutes

Servings: 06

INGREDIENTS

¼ cup Greek yogurt
12 eggs
¼ teaspoon ground black pepper
½ teaspoon salt
1 tablespoon avocado oil
1 cup cherry tomatoes, chopped
1 cup quinoa, cooked
1 cup fresh cilantro, chopped
1 red onion, sliced

STEPS FOR COOKING

1. Boil the eggs in the water within 7 minutes, then cool them in the cold water and peel.
2. Chop the eggs roughly, then put them in the salad bowl.
3. Add Greek yogurt, ground black pepper, salt, avocado oil, tomatoes, quinoa, cilantro, and red onion.
4. Shake the mixture well. Serve.

Scrambled Eggs, Med Style

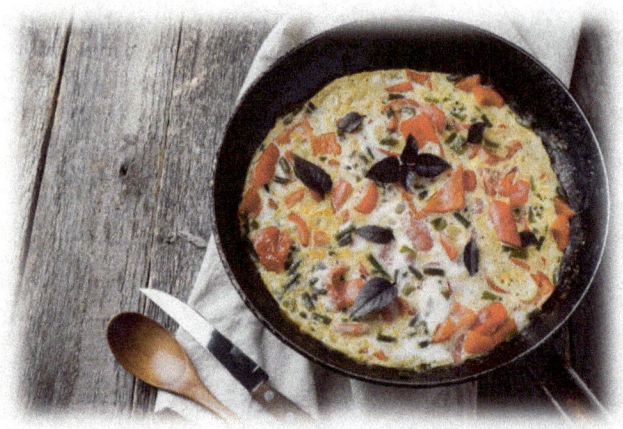

Time required: 10 minutes

Servings: 01

INGREDIENTS

1 tbsp olive oil
2 sliced spring onions
1 sliced yellow pepper
2 tbsp black peppers, de-stoned and sliced
8 quartered cherry tomatoes
1 tbsp capers
0.25 tsp oregano, dried
4 medium eggs
Salt and pepper to season

STEPS FOR COOKING

1. Take a large frying pan and add the oil, heat over a medium temperature.
2. Add the spring onions and peppers and cook until soft.
3. Add the olives, capers, and tomatoes and cook for a further minute.
4. Add the eggs into the pan and use a spoon to scramble them quickly.
5. Add the oregano and season to your liking.
6. Keep scrambling and stirring your eggs until they're as cooked as you like.

Warm Pumpkin Oats

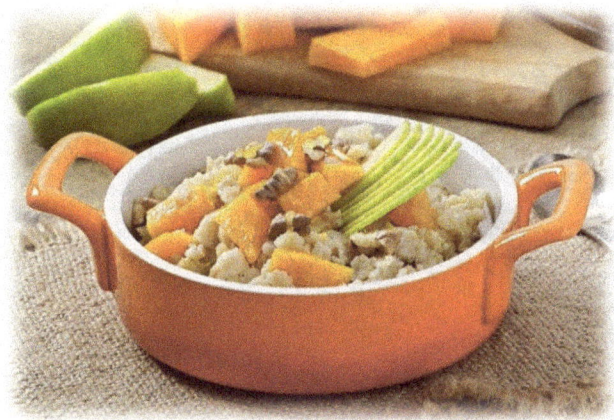

Time required: 20 minutes

Servings: 04

INGREDIENTS

1 cup steel-cut oats
1/4 tsp ground cinnamon
2 1/2 tbsp maple syrup
1 tsp vanilla
2 cups unsweetened almond milk
1/4 cup pumpkin puree
1 cup pumpkin coffee creamer
Pinch of salt

STEPS FOR COOKING

1. Spray instant pot from inside with cooking spray.
2. Add oats, almond milk, coffee creamer, vanilla, and salt into the instant pot and stir well.
3. Seal pot with a lid and select manual and set timer for 10 minutes.
4. Once done, allow to release pressure naturally for 10 minutes then release remaining using quick release. Remove lid.
5. Add remaining ingredients and stir well. Serve and enjoy.

Caprese Breakfast Muffin

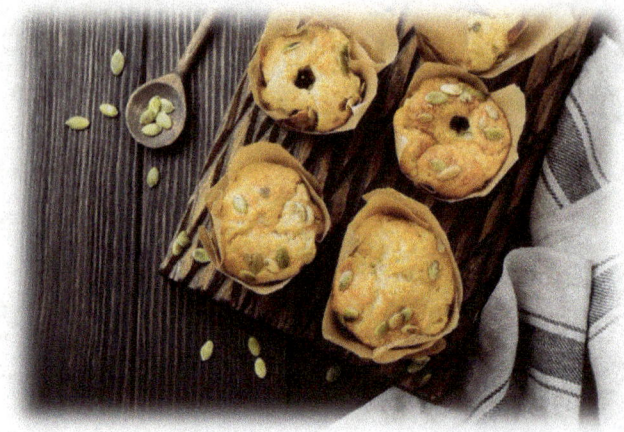

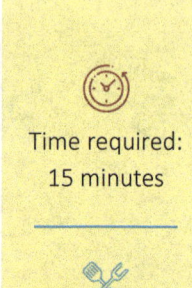

Time required: 15 minutes

Servings: 02

INGREDIENTS

2 wholewheat muffins, split into two

2 chunky slices of fresh tomato

2 egg whites

A handful of spinach leaves

STEPS FOR COOKING

1. Take a non-stick frying pan and cook the egg whites for around 3-4 minutes, until translucent.
2. Meanwhile, toast the muffins to your liking.
3. Split the egg whites between the two bottom sections of the muffins.
4. Add a little spinach to each, a tomato slice to each, and season to your liking.
5. Top with the muffin lid and enjoy.

Buffalo Chicken Chaffle

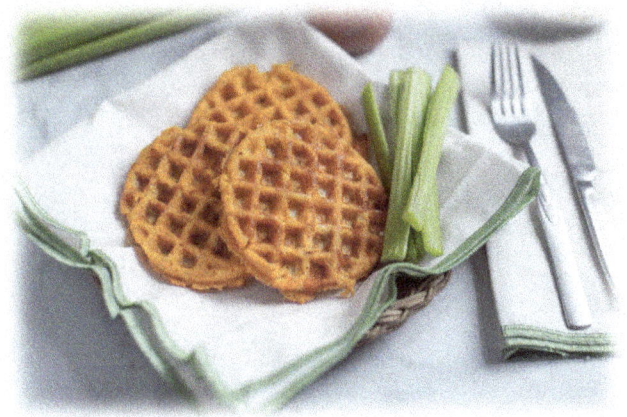

Time required: 20 minutes

Servings: 06

INGREDIENTS

1 Can Valley Fresh Organic Canned Chicken Breast (5 ounces)
2 tbsp Red Hot Wing Sauce
2 oz Cream Cheese softened
4 tbsp Cheddar Cheese shredded
2 tbsp Almond Flour
1 tbsp Nutrition Infoal Yeast
1/2 tsp Baking Powder
1 Egg Yolk Can Use whole egg if no allergy

STEPS FOR COOKING

1. Make flax egg and set aside to rest.
2. Drain liquid from the canned chicken. Mix all the ingredients together. Sprinkle a little cheese on the waffle iron. Let it set for a few seconds before adding 3 T of chicken mixture. (I used a large cookie scooThen add a little more cheese before closing waffle iron. Cook for 5 minutes.
3. Don't open the waffle iron before the time is up or you will have a mess. Remove and let cool before adding a drizzle of hot sauce and ranch dressing.

INGREDIENTS

1 Flax Egg
1 tbsp ground flaxseed
3 tbsp water
*1/4-1/2 Cup Extra Cheese for the waffle iron

STEPS FOR COOKING

Savory Egg Galettes

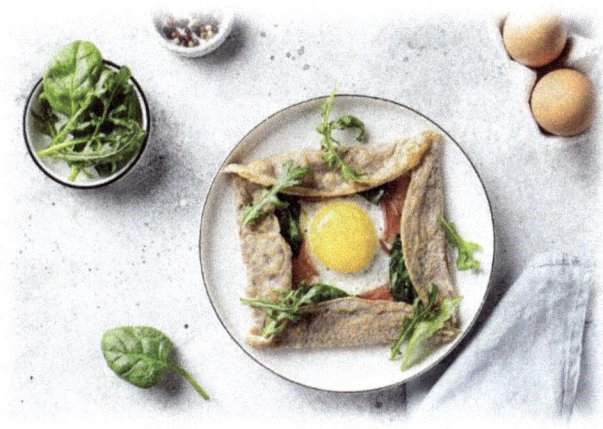

Time required: 45 minutes

Servings: 04

INGREDIENTS

¼ cup white onion, diced
¼ cup bell pepper, chopped
½ teaspoon salt
1 teaspoon chili flakes
2 tablespoons olive oil
1 teaspoon dried dill
6 eggs, beaten
2 tablespoons plain yogurt

STEPS FOR COOKING

1. Mix up onion, bell pepper, salt, then chili flakes in the pan. Add olive oil and dried dill. Sauté the ingredients for 5 minutes.
2. Then pour the beaten eggs into the square baking mold. Add sautéed onion mixture and plain yogurt.
3. Flatten the mixture and bake in the preheated to 360ºF oven for 20 minutes. Cut the meal into galettes.
4. Serve.

Breakfast Cobbler

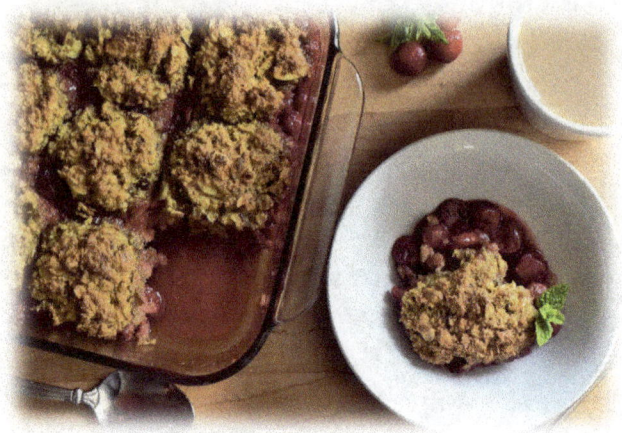

Time required: 22 minutes

Servings: 04

INGREDIENTS

2 lbs apples, cut into chunks
1 1/2 cups water
1/4 tsp nutmeg
1 1/2 tsp cinnamon
1/2 cup dry buckwheat
1/2 cup dates, chopped
Pinch of ground ginger

STEPS FOR COOKING

1. Spray the instant pot from inside with cooking spray, then add all ingredients into the instant pot and stir well.
2. Seal pot with a lid and select manual and set timer for 12 minutes. Once done, release pressure using quick release. Remove lid.
3. Stir and serve.

Carrot Chaffle Cake

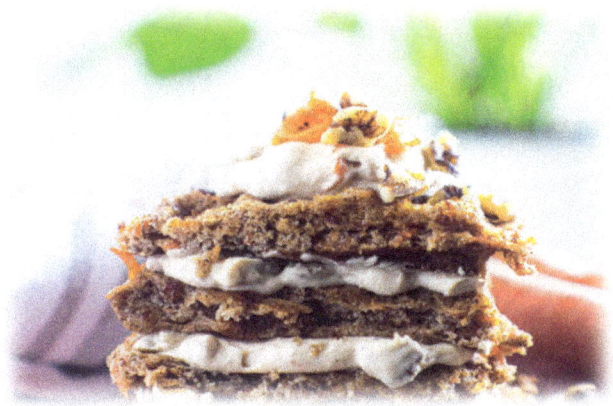

Time required: 10 minutes

Servings: 06

INGREDIENTS

Carrot Chaffle Cake:
1/2 cup carrot shredded
1 egg
2 tbsp butter melted
2 tbsp heavy whipping cream
3/4 cup almond flour
1 tbsp walnuts chopped
2 tbsp powdered sweetener
2 tsp cinnamon
1 tsp pumpkin spice
1 tsp baking powder

Cream Cheese Frosting:

STEPS FOR COOKING

1. Mix your dry ingredients - almond flour, cinnamon, pumpkin spice, baking powder, powdered sweetener, and walnut pieces.
2. Add the wet ingredients- grated carrot, egg, melted butter, heavy cream.
3. Add 3 T batter to preheated mini waffle maker. Cook 2 1/2 - 3 minutes.
4. Mix frosting ingredients together with a hand mixer with whisk attachment until well combined.
5. Stack waffles and add frosting between each layer!

INGREDIENTS

4 oz cream cheese softened

1/4 cup powdered sweetener

1 tsp vanilla extract

1-2 Ttbsp heavy whipping cream

STEPS FOR COOKING

Avocado Wrapped in Bacon

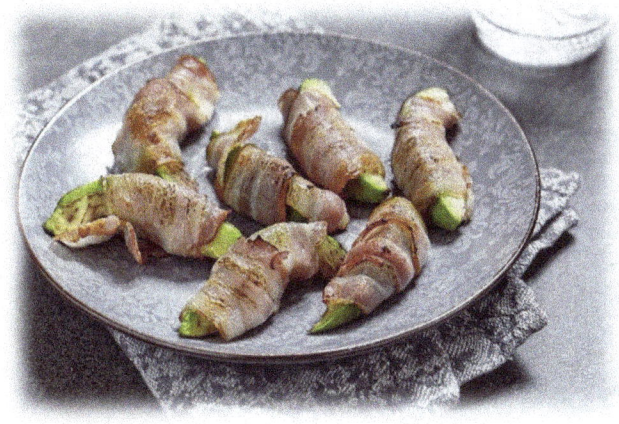

Time required: 25 minutes

Servings: 02

INGREDIENTS

1 avocado
1 egg, cooked
100 g bacon
20 g coconut oil
salt and pepper

STEPS FOR COOKING

1. Wash the avocado and cut it in half. Remove the stone and use a spoon to remove the peel from the avocado.
2. Place the egg in the avocado and close. Layout bacon. Place the avocado on top and coat with it.
3. Heat the oil in a pan and fry the avocado with the bacon in it.

Roasted Veggies

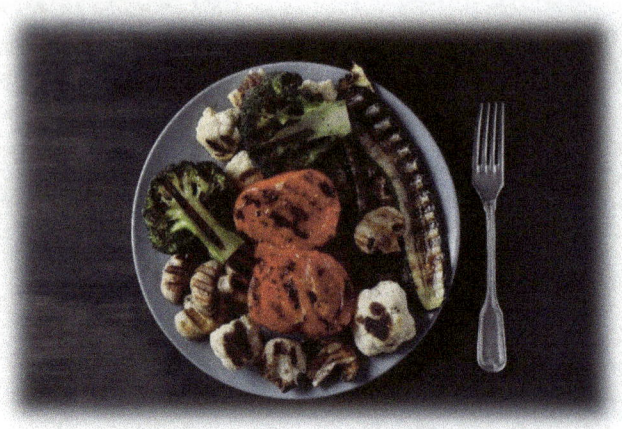

Time required: 30 minutes

Servings: 12

INGREDIENTS

6 cloves garlic
6 tablespoons olive oil
1 fennel bulb, diced
1 zucchini, diced
2 red bell peppers, diced
6 potatoes, large and diced
2 teaspoons sea salt
½ cup balsamic vinegar
¼ cup rosemary, chopped and fresh
2 teaspoons vegetable bouillon powder

STEPS FOR COOKING

1. Heat the oven to 400 F.
2. Get out a baking dish and place your potatoes, fennel, zucchini, garlic, and fennel on a baking dish, drizzling with olive oil.
3. Sprinkle with salt, bouillon powder, and rosemary. Mix well, and then bake at 450 F for thirty to forty minutes.
4. Mix your vinegar into the vegetables before serving.

Mini Keto Pizza

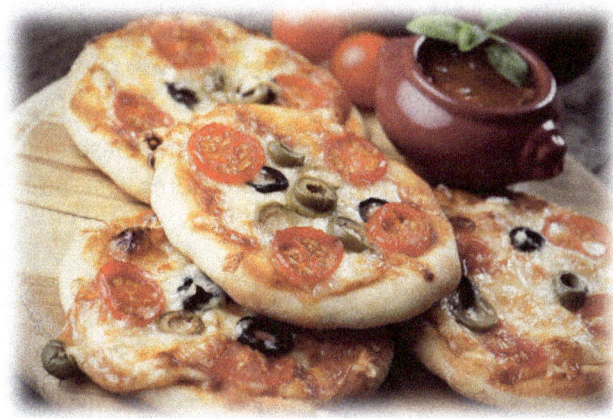

Time required: 15 minutes

Servings: 02

INGREDIENTS

1/2 cup Shredded Mozzarella cheese
1 tablespoons almond flour
1/2 tsp baking powder
1 eggs
1/4 tsp garlic powder
1/4 tsp basil
2 tablespoons low carb pasta sauce
2 tablespoons mozzarella cheese

STEPS FOR COOKING

1. While the waffle maker is heating up, in a bowl mix mozzarella cheese, baking powder, garlic, basis, egg and almond flour.
2. Pour 1/2 the mixture into your mini waffle maker, then cook for 3-5 minutes until your pizza waffle is completely cooked. If you check it and the waffle sticks to the waffle maker let it cook for another minute or two.
3. Next put the remainder of the pizza crust mix into the waffle maker and cook it.
4. Once both pizza crusts are cooked, place them on the baking sheet of your toaster oven.
5. Put 1 tablespoon of low carb pasta sauce on top of each pizza

INGREDIENTS

STEPS FOR COOKING

crust. Sprinkle 1 tablespoon of shredded mozzarella cheese on top of each one.

6. Bake at 350 degrees in the toaster oven for roughly 5 minutes, just until the cheese is melted.

Healthy Tuna Wraps

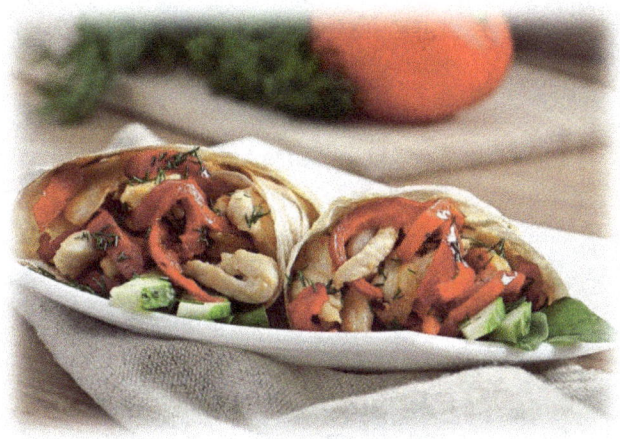

Time required: 20 minutes

Servings: 02

INGREDIENTS

2 egg
2 tbsp mayonnaise
50g green beans, prepared
4 small, sliced gherkins
1 tbsp drained capers
1 can of tuna (spring water)
0.25 tsp mixed herbs (dried)
1 sliced tomato
200g black olives
2 wholewheat tortillas

STEPS FOR COOKING

1. Cook the beans in a pan of boiling water for around 4 minutes.
2. Remove the beans from the water and place them in a bowl of cold water.
3. Drain the beans and place them on one side.
4. Boil the egg in boiling water for 8 minutes, then once cooked, place the egg in cold water to cool.
5. Take a medium bowl and combine the mayonnaise with the herbs, capers, and the gherkin, seasoning well.
6. Add the tuna and combine once more.
7. Remove the egg from the cold water and remove the sheet, cutting it into quarters.

INGREDIENTS	STEPS FOR COOKING
Salt and pepper for seasoning	8. Take the tortillas and add the spinach layers to each one. 9. Add the green beans on top. 10. Add the mixture on top of the tortillas. 11. Add the egg and then the pieces of tomato. 12. Flatten the olives a little and place those on top of the tortillas. 13. Fold the bottom of the wrap inwards and roll-up.

Salmon with a Pesto Crust

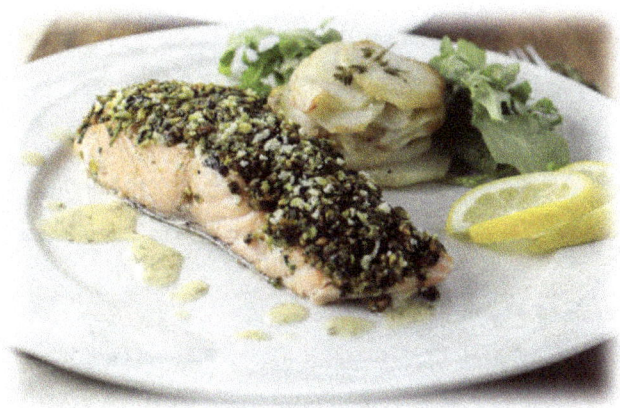

Time required: 30 minutes

Servings: 03

INGREDIENTS

250 g salmon fillet
1 lemon
10 basil leaves
1 clove of garlic
30 g almonds
30 g parmesan cheese
5 tbsp olive oil
200 g green beans
1 tbsp butter
salt and pepper

STEPS FOR COOKING

1. Preheat the oven to 180 ° C top, then bottom heat.
2. Wash basil. Wash the lemon and rub off the peel. Squeeze out the juice. Peel and roughly cut the garlic.
3. Puree the basil, garlic, part of the lemon zest, almonds, parmesan, and olive oil in a blender. Season to taste with salt.
4. Wash the beans and cut the ends, then cook in salted water for 10 minutes.
5. Salt the salmon. Brush with the pesto and bake for 15 minutes.
6. Melt butter in a saucepan. Add the rest of the lemon peel. Roll the beans in it and season with salt, pepper, and lemon juice.

Keto Calamari

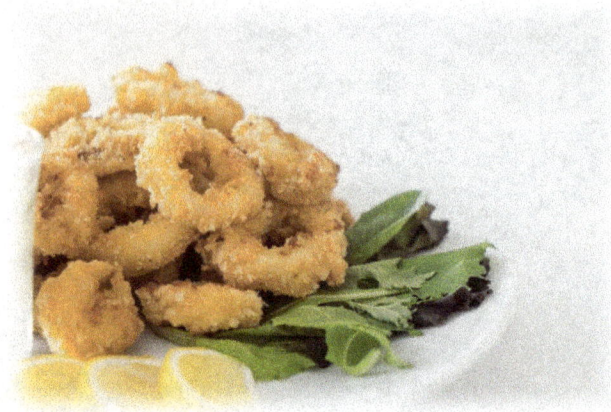

Time required: 15 minutes

Servings: 04

INGREDIENTS

1 lb of squid
3/4 cup coconut flour
1 egg
¼ cup sesame oil
2 Tbsp garlic powder
1 tsp ground cayenne pepper, optional
1 Tbsp onion powder
1 tsp salt
1 tsp pepper
1 cup sweet and spicy garlic and chili sauce

STEPS FOR COOKING

1. Mix all dry ingredients in a large bowl. In a separate container. Beat the egg.
2. Rinse the squid rings and tentacles and dry them with paper towels.
3. Heat the sesame oil in a skillet over high heat.
4. Dip the pieces of squid in the egg and whisk the dry ingredients. Cook in oil for 2-3 min on each side and leave space between pieces of squid.

Courgette Grilled Cheese

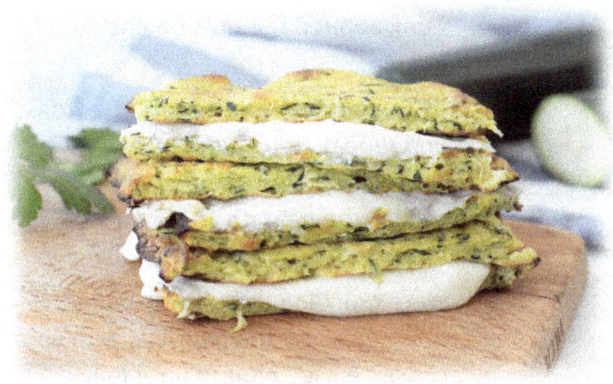

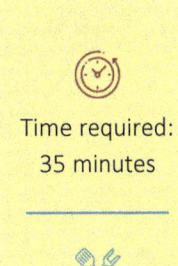

Time required: 35 minutes

Servings: 04

INGREDIENTS

150g grated cheddar or gruyere cheese

20g grated parmesan cheese

30g almond flour

2 courgettes

1 egg

1 spring onion

1 tbsp of butter

STEPS FOR COOKING

1. Grate the courgettes with a box grater or food processor. Chop the spring onions finely.
2. Use a kitchen towel to remove any excess moisture, then press firmly against the courgette to ensure it's as dry as possible, then put away the wet kitchen towel.
3. In a bowl, combine the grated courgette with spring onions, almond flour, parmesan cheese, and egg. Season with salt and pepper.
4. Heat up a pan with butter at medium-high heat.
5. Spoon three tablespoons of your courgette mixture onto the pan. Using your spatula, shape into a rectangle or square so it looks roughly bread-shaped.

INGREDIENTS	STEPS FOR COOKING
	6. Cook about 5 minutes on each until golden. 7. Remove the finished courgette 'toast' and repeat step 5 until all of your courgette mixtures are gone, then reduce the heat on your pan to medium. 8. Place one of your finished courgette toasts back on the pan. Top with your chosen grated cheese until fully covered. Place another courgette toast on top to create a sandwich. 9. Cook for about 1-2 minutes or until the cheese has melted to your liking. 10. Serve and enjoy.

Pork Loin with Cauliflower Mash

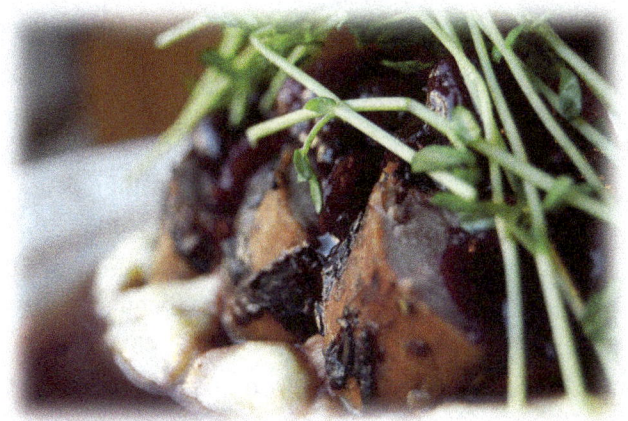

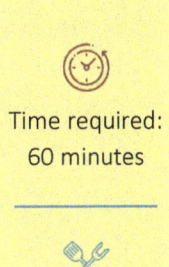

Time required: 60 minutes

Servings: 02

INGREDIENTS

475g pork tenderloin
1 medium cauliflower head
1 tbsp extra virgin olive oil
2 garlic cloves
1 tbsp butter
½ tsp Italian seasoning

STEPS FOR COOKING

1. Preheat the oven to 200°C.
2. In a bowl, combine the olive oil, minced garlic, Italian seasoning, salt, and pepper.
3. Rub or brush each pork loin with olive oil and garlic mixture.
4. Sear your pork loins in a pan over medium-high heat, about 3 minutes on each side.
5. After searing, place your pork loin in the oven and roast for 12-15 minutes, depending on the thickness of your pork.
6. Boil a pot of water.
7. While water heats, cut the cauliflower into small florets.

INGREDIENTS	STEPS FOR COOKING
	8. Add cauliflower to boiling water and cook until tender for about 6-8 minutes. 9. Drain water and keep cauliflower in the warm pot. Add butter, then season with salt and pepper to taste. 10. Mash the buttered cauliflower with a hand-held masher or a blender. Continue until no lumps remain. 11. Remove pork from the oven once its internal temperature has reached 63°C. 12. Serve together and enjoy.

Orange and Fennel Salad

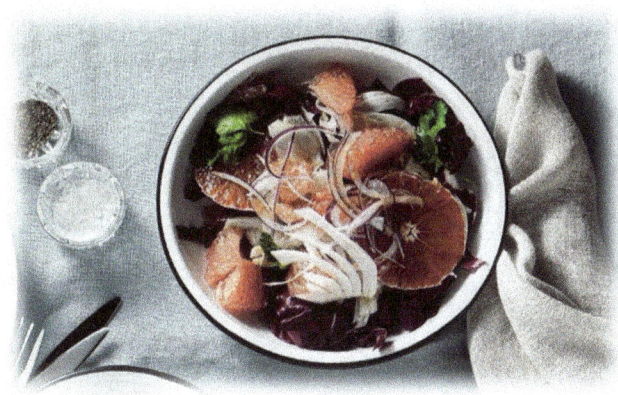

Time required: 10 minutes

Servings: 04

INGREDIENTS

4 tbsp olive oil
2 fennel bulbs
1 large orange
2 tsp sherry vinegar
2 courgettes
1 small lettuce, washed
Juice of half a lemon

STEPS FOR COOKING

1. Remove the peel from the orange and cut it into slices, keeping the juice that runs onto the board.
2. Take the outside of the fennel away and remove the cores.
3. Cut into halves and then smaller pieces.
4. Use a vegetable peeler to cut the courgette into thin slices.
5. Add the loose orange juice, olive oil, and sherry vinegar into a small mixing bowl and combine, adding the lemon juice and combining again.
6. Take a large bowl and combine the orange slices with lettuce, fennel, and courgette.
7. Pour the dressing over the top and combine again.

Guacamole with Coriander and Limes

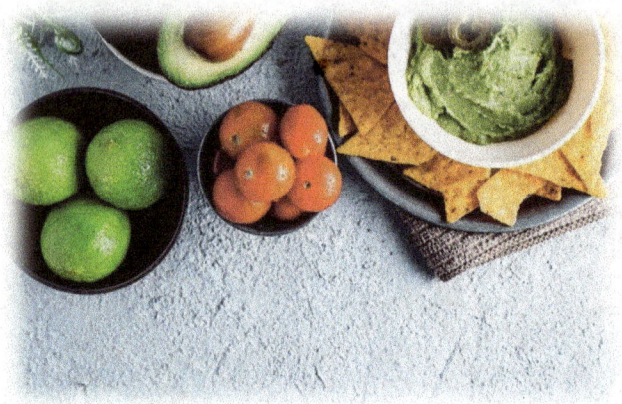

Time required: 25 minutes

Servings: 06

INGREDIENTS

2 avocados

45 g Roma tomatoes, finely diced one chive, minced

4 tablespoons coriander, minced

2 tablespoons lime juice, freshly squeezed

2 teaspoons garlic, finely minced

2 teaspoons jalapeño, finely chopped

½ teaspoon ground coriander

¼ teaspoon cumin, ground salt, to taste

STEPS FOR COOKING

1. Cut avocados lengthwise in half, then remove the pit.
2. Then remove the pulp from the peel, put it in a bowl, and drizzle with the lime juice. Then add salt, cumin, and ground coriander and mash the mixture with a fork until you get a homogeneous dough.
3. Add chives, tomatoes, jalapeños, garlic, and chopped cilantro, stir well, and season again with salt if necessary.

Caponata Lamb

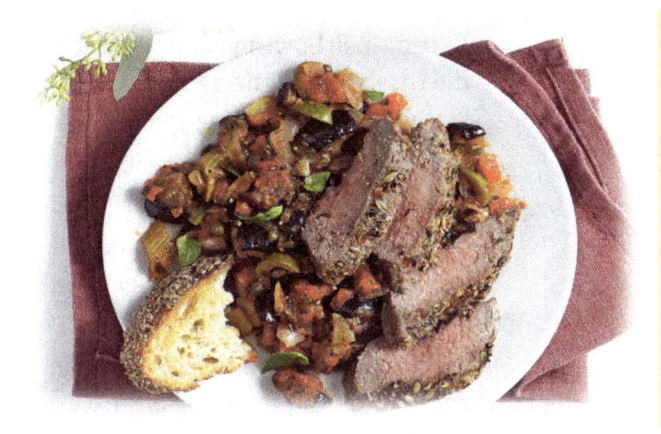

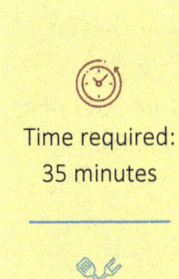

Time required: 35 minutes

Servings: 02

INGREDIENTS

2 tsp olive oil, plus 1 extra tsp for the lamb

250g lamb fillet, all fat removed

3 cloves of garlic

1 sliced red onion

1 sliced aubergine

1 sliced green pepper

6 halved, pitted olives

1 carton of passata

2 tbsp rinsed capers

1 tsp balsamic vinegar

2 tsp chopped rosemary

STEPS FOR COOKING

1. Take two of the garlic cloves and slice them finely, grate the other one, and put it aside.
2. Take a large frying pan and add the oil over medium heat.
3. Add the onion and cook for 5 minutes, then the aubergine and cook for another 5 minutes.
4. Add the passata to the pan, then the capers, half the rosemary, the olives, and the balsamic vinegar, combining well.
5. Cover the pan and cook for 15 minutes, stirring every few minutes.
6. Heat your oven to 170 C.
7. Take a medium saucepan and boil the potatoes for 10 minutes, raining once cooked.

INGREDIENTS	STEPS FOR COOKING
4 halved new potatoes *1 bag of baby spinach*	8. Take a small bowl and add the rest of the rosemary, a little pepper, and the grated garlic, combining well. 9. Rub the mixture over the lamb, ensuring it is fully coated. 10. Take a small roasting tin and add the lamb inside, placing it in the oven for 20 minutes. 11. Meanwhile, add the spinach to a pan and all it to wilt, removing any excess water. 12. Add the rest of the garlic mixture to the passata pan and combine. 13. Serve the mixture alongside the lamb.

Grilled Shrimp Salad

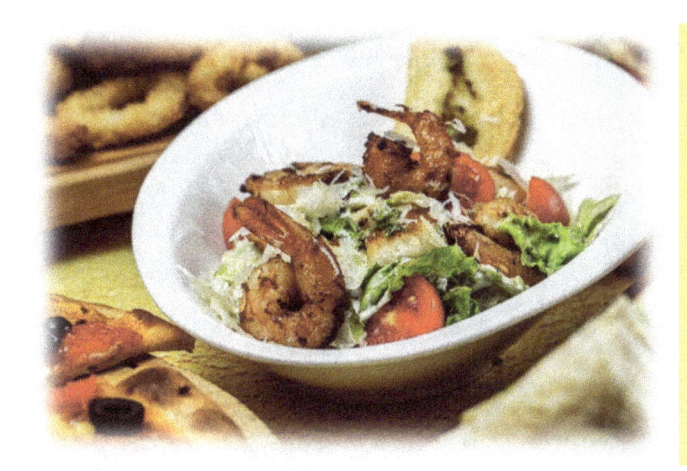

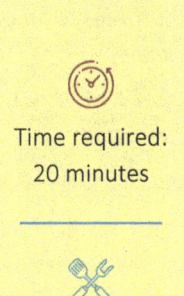

Time required: 20 minutes

Servings: 02

INGREDIENTS

1 pound of Large Deveined Shrimp

3 Zucchini

2 pounds of Salad Mixture (Containing Radicchio, Butter Lettuce, and Endive)

1 bunch of Asparagus

1 teaspoon of Dijon Mustard

2 tablespoons of Fresh Chopped Basil

1 Avocado

3/4 cup of Extra-Virgin Olive Oil

2 teaspoons of Minced Garlic

STEPS FOR COOKING

1. Combine your mustard, olive oil, garlic, red wine vinegar, lime juice, and basil. Marinate your shrimp in half of your vinaigrette mixture for 30 minutes.
2. Place your shrimp on skewers. Slice your zucchini lengthwise. Chop the woody ends off of your asparagus.
3. Heat up your grill. Place your shrimp, zucchini, and asparagus on your grill, and cook until finished.
4. Chop your zucchini into bite-sized pieces. Place your salad mixture greens in a bowl. Dice your avocado and add it to your greens.
5. Add your shrimp and vegetables from off your grill. Drizzle with your remaining vinaigrette mixture.

INGREDIENTS	STEPS FOR COOKING
1 tablespoon of Lime Juice *1/4 cup of Red Wine Vinegar*	6. Serve!

Mediterranean Stuffed Tomatoes

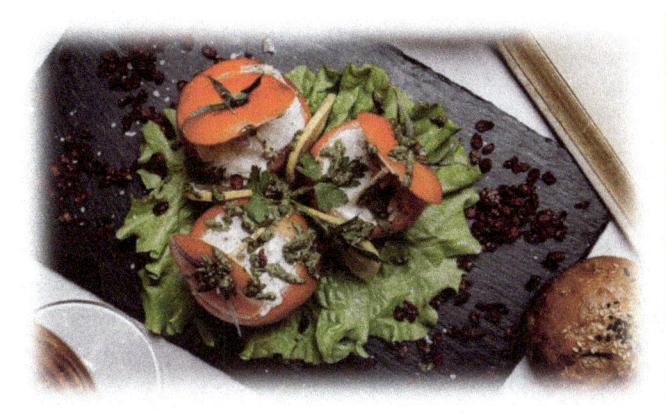

Time required: 25 minutes

Servings: 04

INGREDIENTS

2 Large Tomatoes

1/2 cup of Packaged Garlic Croutons

2 tablespoons of Reduced-Fat Vinaigrette

1/4 cup of Crumbled Goat Cheese

2 tablespoons of Chopped Fresh Thyme

1/4 cup of Sliced and Pitted Olives

STEPS FOR COOKING

1. Preheat your broiler.
2. Cut your tomatoes in half crosswise. Use your finger to push out and discard any seeds. Use your paring knife to cut out all the pulp, leaving 2 shells. Chop your pulp, and transfer it to your medium-sized bowl. Place your hollowed tomatoes, cut sides down, on your paper towel. Drain for approximately 5 minutes. Add your goat cheese, croutons, dressing, olives, and thyme to your pulp. Mix it all together well. Mound your mixture into your hollowed tomatoes.
3. Place your tomatoes on your broiler pan or baking sheet. Broil approximately 4 to 5-inches from the heat until hot and your cheese melts. Should take approximately 5 minutes.
4. Serve!

Cheesy Spinach Chicken

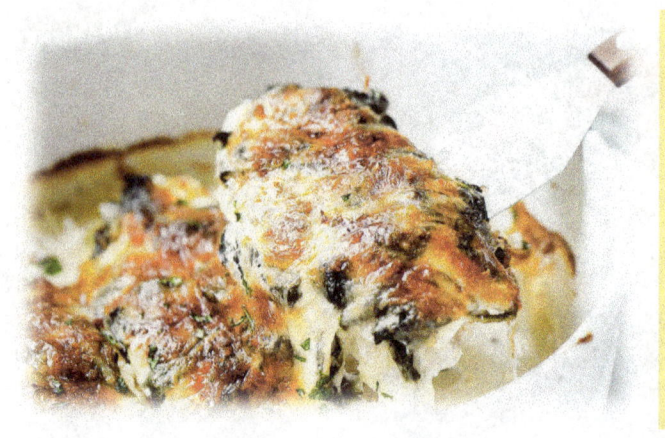

Time required: 60 minutes

Servings: 04

INGREDIENTS

1 tbsp olive oil
85g cream cheese
4 chicken breasts
1 sliced onion
20 cherry tomatoes
200g pre-thawed frozen chicken, chopped
500g sliced potato
4 sliced garlic cloves
8 chopped black olives
A pinch of grated nutmeg

STEPS FOR COOKING

1. Preheat the oven to 220 C.
2. Take a large baking sheet and line it with baking parchment.
3. Take a mixing bowl and add the onion, covering over with boiling water.
4. Leave the bowl to soak for 15 minutes.
5. Take another bowl and add the spinach, cheese, and nutmeg and combine well.
6. Spread the mixture over the chicken breasts.
7. Place the tomatoes over the top.
8. Take the onion and drain the water.
9. Place the potatoes, onion, garlic, oil, and olives into another mixing bowl and season well, tossing to coat.

INGREDIENTS	STEPS FOR COOKING
	10. Place the potatoes onto the parchment and flatten out.
	11. Place in the oven for 25 minutes.
	12. Once cooked, arrange the potatoes into four piles and place a chicken breast on top of each one.
	13. Place back into the oven for another 20 minutes, making sure that the chicken is fully cooked.

Simple Tomato Soup

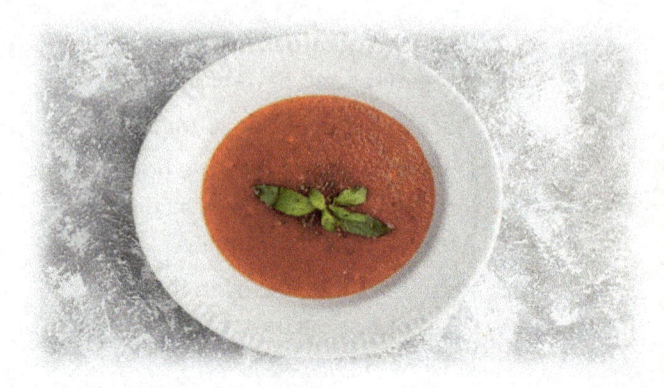

Time required: 15 minutes

Servings: 04

INGREDIENTS

1 quart canned tomato soup

4 tablespoons ghee

¼ cup olive oil

¼ cup red hot sauce

2 tablespoons apple cider vinegar

Salt and black pepper to the taste

1 teaspoon oregano, dried

2 teaspoon turmeric, ground

8 bacon strips, cooked and crumbled

A handful of green onions, chopped

A handful of basil leaves, chopped

STEPS FOR COOKING

1. Put tomato soup in a pot and heat up over medium heat.
2. Add olive oil, ghee, hot sauce, vinegar, salt, pepper, turmeric, and oregano, stir and simmer for 5 minutes.
3. Take off heat, divide the soup into bowls, top with bacon crumbles, basil, and green onions.
4. Enjoy!

Chicken and Shrimp

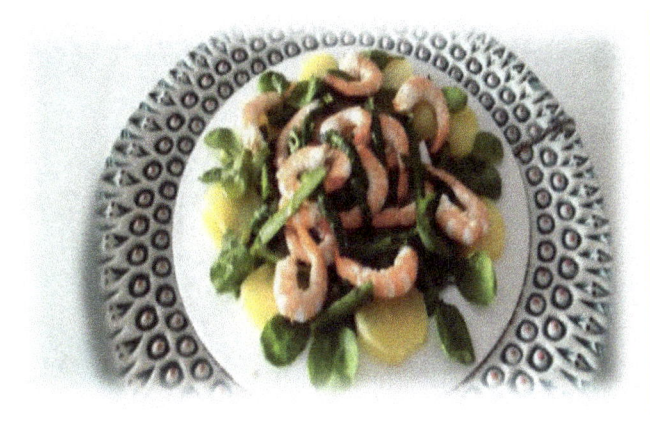

Time required: 30 minutes

Servings: 02

INGREDIENTS

- 20 shrimp, raw, peeled, and deveined
- 2 chicken breasts, boneless and skinless
- 2 handfuls spinach leaves
- ½ pound mushrooms, roughly chopped
- Salt and black pepper to the taste
- ¼ cup mayonnaise
- 2 tablespoons sriracha
- 2 teaspoons lime juice

STEPS FOR COOKING

1. Heat up a pan with the oil over medium-high heat, add chicken breasts, season with salt, pepper, red pepper, and garlic powder, cook for 8 minutes, flip and cook for 6 minutes more.
2. Add mushrooms, more salt, and pepper, and cook for a few minutes.
3. Heat up another pan, add shrimp, sriracha, paprika, xantham, and mayo, then stir and cook until shrimp turn pink.
4. Take off heat, add lime juice, then stir everything.
5. Divide spinach on plates, chicken, and mushroom, top with shrimp mix, garnish with green onions.
6. Serve and enjoy!

INGREDIENTS

1 tablespoon coconut oil

½ teaspoon red pepper, crushed

1 teaspoon garlic powder

½ teaspoon paprika

¼ teaspoon xantham gum

1 green onion stalk, chopped

STEPS FOR COOKING

Warming Fish Stew

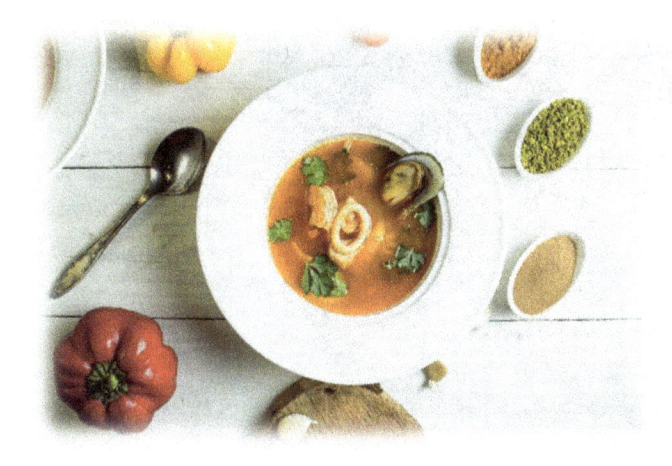

Time required: 35 minutes

Servings: 02

INGREDIENTS

1 tbsp olive oil
85g shelled king prawns (raw)
2 fillets of pollock, skinless and cut into large chunks
500ml cooked fish stock (hot)
1 tsp fennel seeds
2 diced celery sticks
2 diced carrots
2 chopped garlic cloves
2 sliced leeks
1 can of chopped tomatoes

STEPS FOR COOKING

1. Take a large pan and add the oil over medium heat.
2. Add the carrots, celery, garlic, and fennel seeds, cooking for 5 minutes, until softened.
3. Add the leeks, the stock, and the tomatoes and combine.
4. Cover the pan and bring to the boil, then turn down to a simmer for around 20 minutes. The sauce should have thickened and the vegetables should be soft.
5. Add the pollock and the prawns and cook for another 2 minutes, ensuring that the prawns are cooked properly before serving.

Tuscan Chicken Skillet

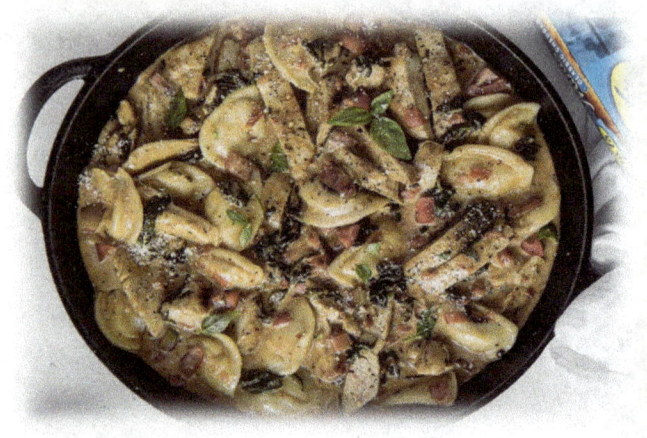

Time required: 35 minutes

Servings: 04

INGREDIENTS

5 ounces of Chicken Breast Tenderloin

2 teaspoons of Olive Oil

7 ounces of Diced Canned Tomatoes

1/4 cup of Sun-Dried Tomatoes, sliced

1/4 teaspoon of Oregano

2 tablespoons of Diced Onion

1/8 teaspoon of thyme

3 ounces of Button Mushrooms, sliced

1 clove of Minced Garlic

STEPS FOR COOKING

1. Season your chicken with salt and pepper. Heat 1 tablespoon of your olive oil in a large-sized sauté pan or cast-iron skillet over medium-high heat, then add your chicken and brown for approximately 3 minutes on each side.

2. Remove your chicken and set it to the side on your plate. Add your remaining tablespoon of olive oil to your pan. Add your sliced mushrooms in a single layer and brown, working in batches, a few minutes per side. Remove from your pan and set to the side.

3. Add your onion and sauté for approximately 3 minutes. Add your garlic and sun-dried tomatoes. Sauté for about 2 minutes. Stir in your

INGREDIENTS

3 1/2 ounces of Cannellini Beans, drained and rinsed

1 teaspoon of Sugar

1/4 teaspoon of Chili Flakes

1/4 teaspoon of Sea Salt

1/4 teaspoon of Freshly Ground Pepper Parsley, for garnish

STEPS FOR COOKING

oregano, beans, thyme, diced tomatoes, and sugar.

4. Transfer your chicken back to your pan and spoon some of your sauce and vegetables over top of your chicken. Cook, covered, on your stovetop until your chicken is cooked through and the sauce is bubbling. Should take about 10 minutes. Return your mushrooms to the pan. Add your salt and pepper as needed. Garnish with your parsley.
5. Serve!

Caprese Salad

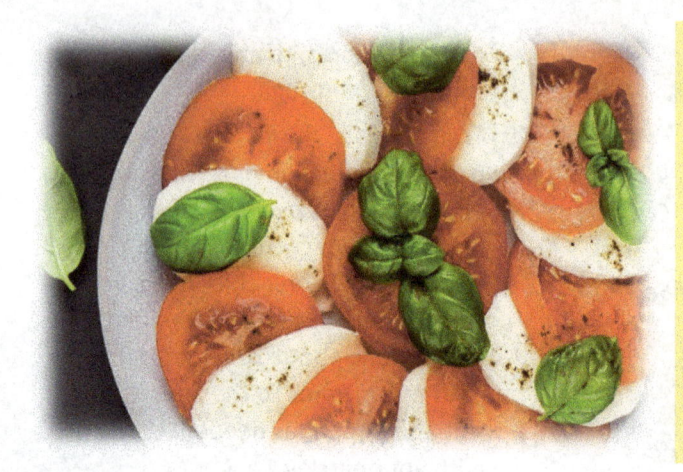

Time required: 10 minutes

Servings: 02

INGREDIENTS

½ pound mozzarella cheese, sliced

1 tomato, sliced

Salt and black pepper to the taste

4 basil leaves, torn

1 tablespoon balsamic vinegar

1 tablespoon olive oil

STEPS FOR COOKING

1. Alternate tomato and mozzarella slices on 2 plates, then sprinkle salt, pepper, drizzle vinegar, and olive oil.
2. Sprinkle basil leaves at the end.
3. Serve and enjoy!

Spanish Chilled Soup

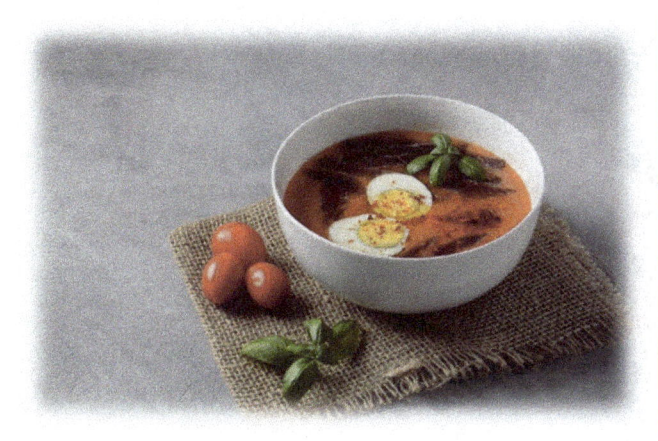

Time required: 20 minutes

Servings: 04

INGREDIENTS

3 tbsp cider vinegar
75ml olive oil
8 large, chopped tomatoes
3 chopped garlic cloves
1 chopped green pepper, seeds removed
2 slices of wholewheat bread
Half a chopped red onion
1 egg, boiled
50g chopped Serrano ham
100ml water

STEPS FOR COOKING

1. Take a small dish and soak the bread in water for around 30 seconds.
2. Turn the bread over and soak for another 30 seconds on the other side.
3. Take a food processor and add the bread, green pepper, olive oil, tomatoes, and garlic, blitzing until smooth.
4. Add the cider vinegar, a little salt, and 100ml of water.
5. Blitz once more until everything is combined and smooth.
6. Place the soup in the refrigerator for around an hour.
7. When you're ready to serve, drizzle with a small amount of olive oil and add the ham, onion, and sliced boiled egg on top.

Skinny Bruschetta Chicken

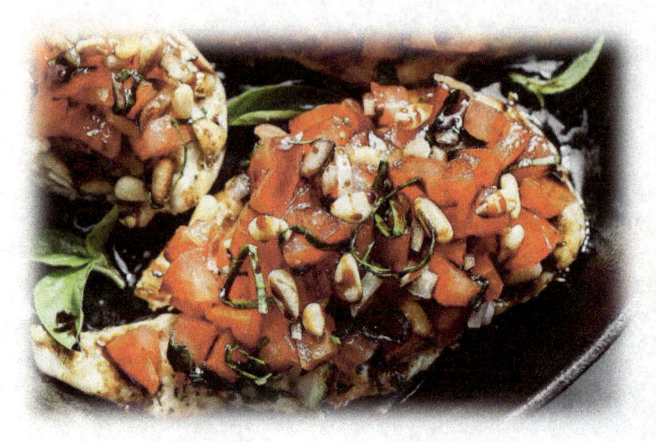

Time required: 50 minutes

Servings: 04

INGREDIENTS

4 Chicken Breasts
1 clove of Minced Garlic
1 teaspoon of Balsamic Vinegar
1 teaspoon of Olive Oil
5 Small Tomatoes, Chopped
1/8 teaspoon of Sea Salt
A handful of Chopped Basil

STEPS FOR COOKING

1. Preheat your oven to 375 degrees. Sprinkle some salt and pepper over top. Cover and bake for approximately 35 to 40 minutes until the juices run clear.
2. Combine your chopped tomatoes, olive oil, garlic, balsamic vinegar, sea salt, and basil in your bowl. Spoon over top of your chicken.
3. Serve!

Easy Parmesan Crusted Tilapia

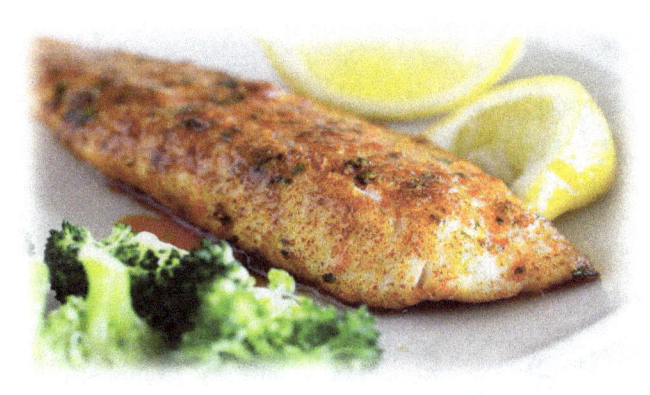

Time required: 20 minutes

Servings: 04

INGREDIENTS

3/4 cup grated Parmesan cheese

1/3 teaspoon salt

1/4 teaspoon red pepper flakes, crushed

1 pound tilapia fillets, cut into 4 servings

1/3 teaspoon ground black pepper

2 tablespoons olive oil

STEPS FOR COOKING

1. Start with seasoning the fish fillets with salt, black pepper, and red pepper flakes.
2. Now, brush tilapia fillets with olive oil; press them into the Parmesan cheese.
3. Put fish fillets on a foil-lined baking sheet. Bake for approximately 10 minutes or until fish fillets is opaque.

Crabmeat, Prosciutto, and Vegetable Delight

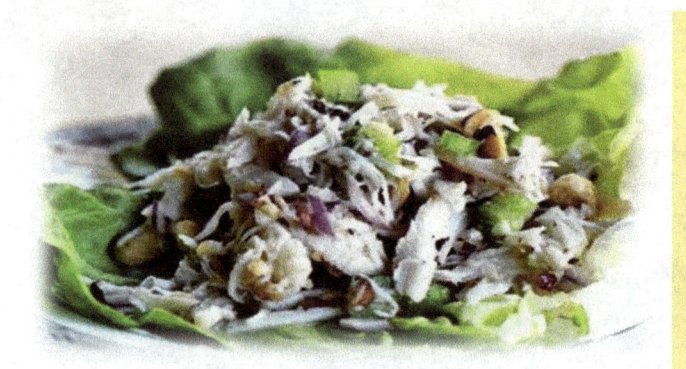

Time required: 10 minutes

Servings: 04

INGREDIENTS

1 tablespoon tahini
1/2 lemon, zested and juiced
3 tablespoons olive oil
2 cans lump crabmeat, drained
1/2 cup fresh Italian parsley, chopped
2 ounces thinly sliced prosciutto, chopped
10 cherry tomato, halved
Coarse salt and ground black pepper
4 cups baby spinach
10 ripe olives, pitted and halved

STEPS FOR COOKING

1. In a small-sized mixing bowl, whisk the lemon zest, oil, tahini, lemon juice, salt, and pepper.
2. In a salad container, gently toss the crabmeat with spinach, prosciutto, cherry tomatoes, and olives. Drizzle with the prepared dressing and toss to merge.
3. Finally, serve garnished with fresh parsley in individual salad bowls.

Fully Stuffed Peppers

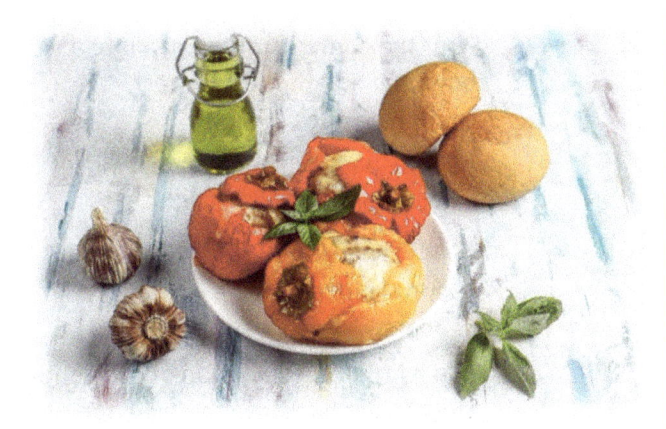

Time required: 45 minutes

Servings: 02

INGREDIENTS

1 tbsp olive oil
50g whole grain rice
1 red pepper
1 yellow pepper
1 sliced onion
1 diced courgette
2 crushed garlic cloves
75g cherry tomatoes, cut into halves
Zest of half an orange
1 tsp cumin
1 tsp coriander, ground
3 tbsp flat leave parsley, chopped

STEPS FOR COOKING

1. Preheat the oven to 200 C.
2. Cook the rice according to instructions and drain well.
3. Take the red and yellow pepper and cut into halves, straight down the middle. Cut out the seeds.
4. Cover a baking tray with parchment paper and arrange the peppers on top, with the open side upwards.
5. Place into the oven for 15 minutes.
6. Take a large frying pan and add the oil over medium heat.
7. Cook the courgette and onions until soft and brown, stirring every so often.
8. Add the garlic, tomatoes, coriander, and cumin and combine well.
9. Cook for one minute.

INGREDIENTS

100g goat's cheese, cut into chunks

Salt and pepper for seasoning

STEPS FOR COOKING

10. Pour the contents of the pan into a bowl and add the orange zest, combining once more.
11. Add the parsley and the cooked rice and combine.
12. Season and combine again.
13. Spoon the rice mixture into the peppers.
14. Add a little cheese on top of each one and place it back into the oven for 10 minutes.

Scallops Provencal

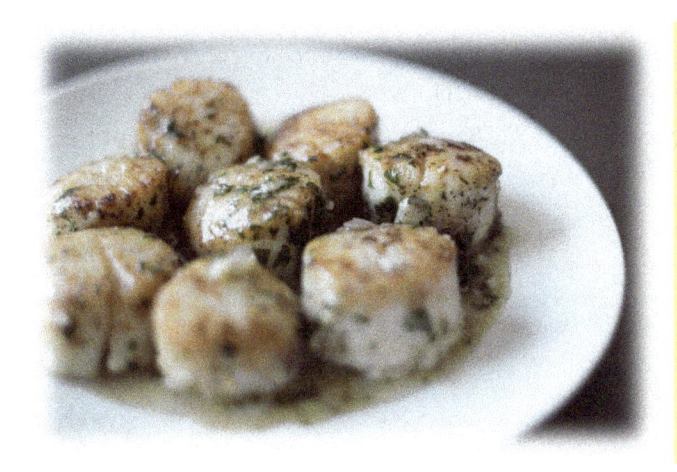

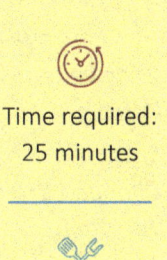

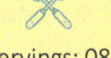

Time required: 25 minutes

Servings: 08

INGREDIENTS

1 pound of Sea Scallops, rinsed and drained

2 tablespoons of Butter

1/4 pound of Frozen Small Cooked Shrimp

1/2 pound of Mushrooms, Thinly Sliced

1 Small Onion, finely chopped

2 Medium Tomatoes, peeled and chopped

1 clove of Minced Garlic

STEPS FOR COOKING

1. Heat your butter in a large-sized skillet over medium-high heat. Without crowding, lightly your brown scallops in batches. Remove your scallops to individual casseroles or lightly buttered baking shells.

2. Stir your onion and mushrooms into your skillet, and cook until your onion is soft and begins to brown.

3. Stir in your garlic, wine, tomatoes, ketchup, rosemary, salt, tarragon, and white pepper, then bring to a boil. Cover, reduce heat to low and simmer for approximately 15 minutes. Uncover, and cook until thick. Should take about 3 minutes. Mix in your shrimp and vinegar.

4. Preheat your oven to 400 degrees.

INGREDIENTS

1/4 teaspoon of Dried Rosemary

2 tablespoons of Ketchup

1/2 teaspoon of Chopped Dried Tarragon

2 teaspoons of White Wine Vinegar

1/2 teaspoon of Salt

Pinch of White Pepper

Chopped Fresh Parsley, for Garnish

1/4 cup of Dry White Wine (Optional)

STEPS FOR COOKING

5. Spoon your sauce evenly over your scallops.
6. Bake in your preheated oven until sauce bubbles and begins to brown at the edges. Should take about 10 minutes. Sprinkle parsley over tops.
7. Serve!

Roasted Lemon Asparagus

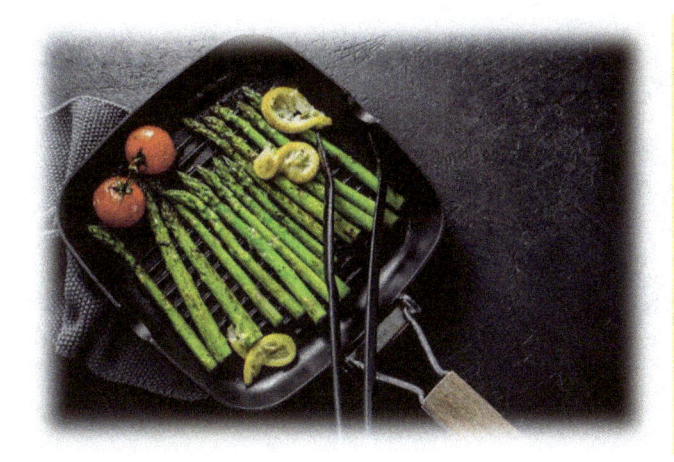

Time required: 20 minutes

Servings: 03

INGREDIENTS

1 tbsp. chopped oregano,
Salt
3 tsp. Avocado oil
1 bunch trimmed asparagus
Lemon juice
Black pepper

STEPS FOR COOKING

1. Season the asparagus then align in a baking tray. Sprinkle with olive oil, oregano, and lemon juice. Toss to coat evenly.
2. Set the oven for 10 minutes at 450 0F then allow to bake.
3. Serve hot.

Sicilian Marinated Olives

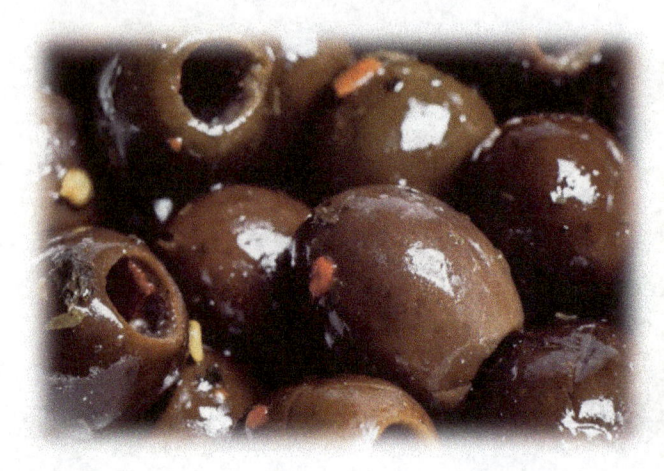

Time required: 40 minutes

Servings: 08

INGREDIENTS

1 Medium Chopped Celery Stalk

1 1/2 cup of Unpitted Green Olives

3 tablespoons of Chopped Flat-Leaf Parsley

1 teaspoon of White-Wine Vinegar

1 Small Fresh Red or Green Chile Pepper, sliced thin

2 tablespoons of Extra-Virgin Olive Oil

1/8 teaspoon of Dried Oregano

STEPS FOR COOKING

1. Rinse your olives in a colander, tossing them gently under some running water, then dry using your kitchen towel. Transfer to your bowl. Add your oil and gently toss to coat.
2. Add your garlic, celery, 2 tablespoons of parsley, chile, and vinegar. Toss again to combine. Let your olives stand at room temperature for approximately 30 minutes.
3. Transfer to your serving platter and sprinkle with your remaining 1 tablespoon of parsley and oregano. You want to crumble the oregano with your fingers to help bring out the flavor.
4. Serve!

Fig and Anise Ice Cream

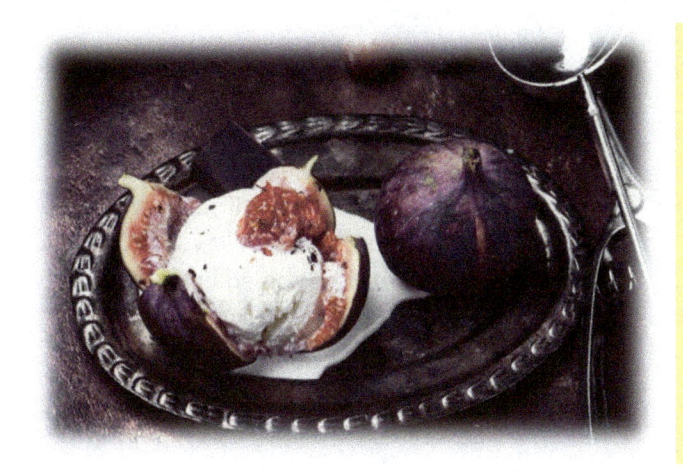

Time required: 30 minutes

Servings: 12

INGREDIENTS

1 1/2 pound of Ripe Figs, unpeeled and stems removed
1 cup of Creme Fraiche
3 Large Eggs, separated
2 cups of Cream
1/3 cup of Honey
1/3 cup + 2 tablespoons of Sugar
1 teaspoon of Aniseed

STEPS FOR COOKING

1. Puree your figs in your food processor or blender. Transfer your puree to your 10-inch skillet with 1/3 cup of sugar.
2. Cook over medium heat, stirring often to prevent any sticking until your figs have thickened into a jam. Should take about 30 minutes.
3. In your saucepan, heat your honey, cream, and aniseed over medium heat. Bring to a boil, stirring to dissolve your honey. Whisk a little of your hot cream into your egg yolks, and then whisk them back into your pan. Cook over low heat, stirring constantly until your mixture thickens and coats your spoon. Immediately transfer to your bowl.

INGREDIENTS	STEPS FOR COOKING
	4. Stir in your fig puree and crème fraîche and chill thoroughly. Whisk your egg whites until foamy. Add your remaining 2 tablespoons of sugar and continue beating until you have formed soft peaks. Fold your egg whites into the cooled fig puree, and freeze in your ice cream maker following your manufacturer's instructions. 5. Serve!

Healthier Brownies

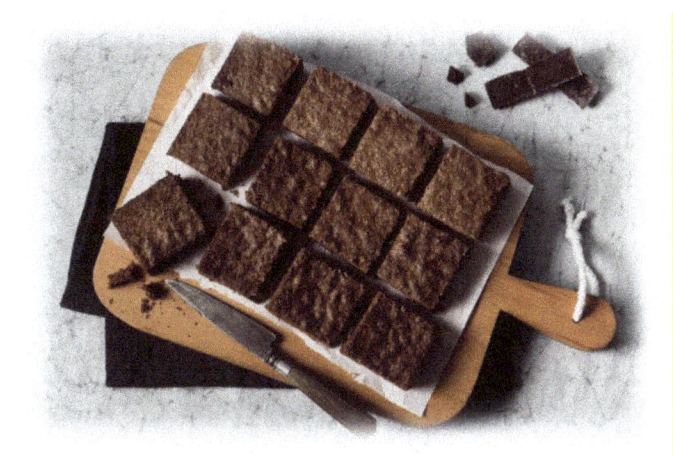

Time required: 45 minutes

Servings: 08

INGREDIENTS

59ml olive oil
32g Greek yogurt
2 eggs
1 tsp vanilla extract
64g flour
96g sugar
0.5 tsp baking powder
Pinch of salt
50g cocoa powder
20g chopped walnuts

STEPS FOR COOKING

1. Preheat your oven to 220 C.
2. Take a mixing bowl and add the sugar and olive oil, mixing everything together well.
3. Add the vanilla and mix again.
4. Take a small mixing bowl and add the eggs, beating until smooth.
5. Add the other mixture and combine.
6. Pour the yogurt into the mixture and combine again.
7. Take another bowl and add the cocoa powder, flour, baking powder, and salt, combining.
8. Add to the other mixture and combine again.
9. Add the nuts and combine once more.

INGREDIENTS	STEPS FOR COOKING
	10. Take a square 9" baking tin and line it with parchment paper.
11. Pour the mixture into the pan and smooth the top, then place in the oven and cook for 25 minutes.
12. Once cooled, cut into squares.

Honey Yogurt with Balsamic Berries

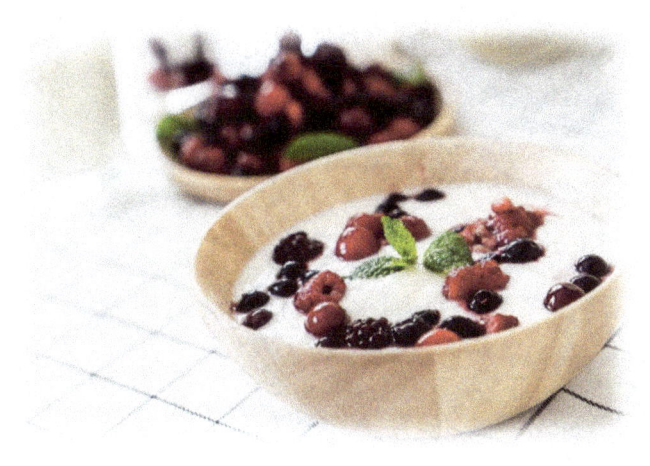

Time required: 15 minutes

Servings: 04

INGREDIENTS

8 quartered strawberries
1 tbsp balsamic vinegar
128g raspberries
128g blueberries
2 tsp honey
157ml Greek yogurt

STEPS FOR COOKING

1. Take a large bowl and add the berries and balsamic vinegar.
2. Combine, then allow to rest for 10 minutes.
3. Take a small bowl and add the honey and yogurt, combining well.
4. Take four serving bowls and divide the berries equally between them.
5. Place a large serving of the yogurt on top of each one.

Ricotta Cake

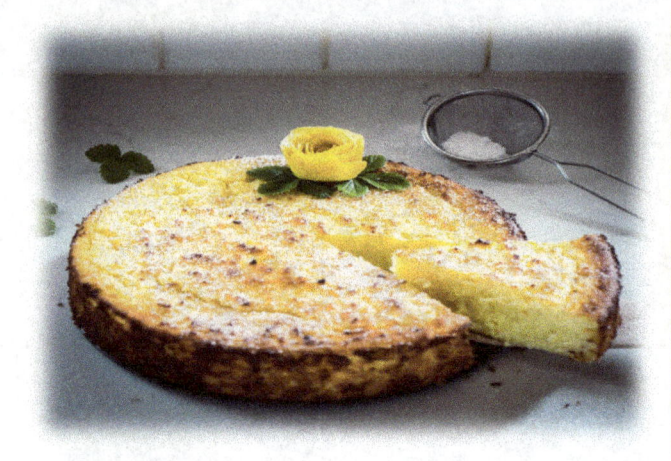

Time required: 70 minutes

Servings: 04

INGREDIENTS

8 Eggs
1/2 pound of Sugar
3 pounds of Fresh Ricotta Cheese
Zest of 1 Orange
Zest of 1 Lemon
Butter

STEPS FOR COOKING

1. In your bowl mix together all your ingredients.
2. Coat your bottom and sides of your 9-inch springform pan with butter.
3. Pour your mix into your springform pan.
4. Bake for approximately 30 minutes at 425 degrees. Continue baking for an additional 40 minutes at 380 degrees.
5. Allow it to cool.
6. Serve!

Coco Macaroons

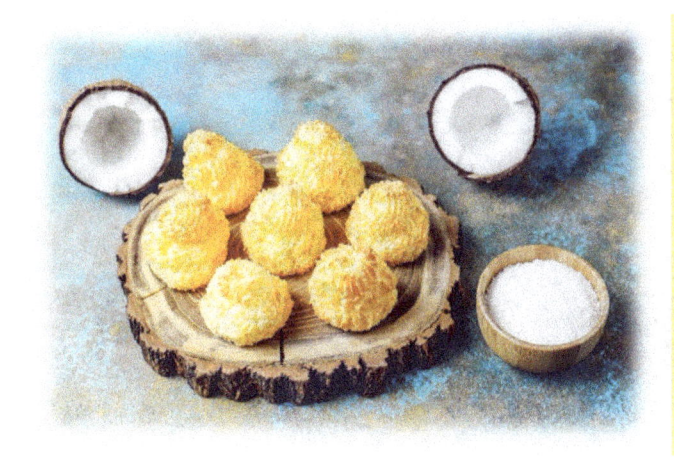

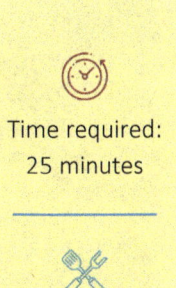

Time required: 25 minutes

Servings: 20

INGREDIENTS

1/3 cup sweetener

3 eggs whites, whipped

2 cups coconut, finely shredded

STEPS FOR COOKING

1. Preheat your oven to 160C and prepare the baking sheet with parchment paper.
2. Carefully add coconut and sweetener to the whipped white eggs. Make about 20 small balls with the dough.
3. Place the balls in the baking sheet and press each one to form a cookie. Bake for approx. 20 minutes or until golden brown.
4. Serve and enjoy!

Caramel Cookies

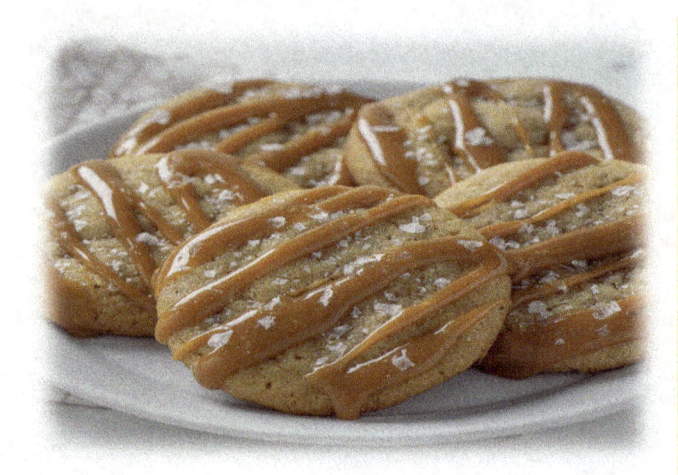

Time required: 25 minutes

Servings: 08

INGREDIENTS

12 drops caramel flavoring

1 cup almond flour, finely ground

¼ cup brown sweetener

¼ cup butter softened

¼ cup cashews shredded

A pinch of salt

STEPS FOR COOKING

1. Preheat your oven to 325°F and prepare the baking sheet with parchment paper.
2. Add all the ingredients to a small mixing bowl and stir until well combined, then wrap the dough in the parchment paper and roll it into a cylinder.
3. Cut the dough into thin slices, then place them on a baking sheet. Bake for approx. 10-15 minutes or until golden brown.
4. Serve and enjoy!

Pecans with Caramel

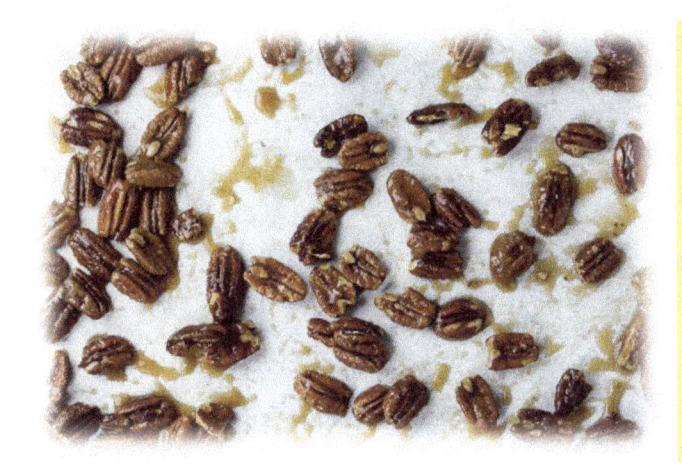

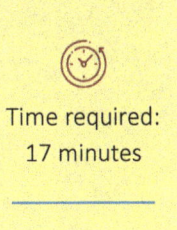

Time required: 17 minutes

Servings: 06

INGREDIENTS

1 tsp vanilla extract
½ cup brown sweetener
¼ cup butter
1 ½ cup pecan halves

STEPS FOR COOKING

1. In a small saucepan over low heat melt the butter, then add the sweetener and stir constantly.
2. Add one tsp of vanilla and mix well.
3. Simmer for 10 minutes until it begins to thicken, then remove from heat and add the pecans to the pot.
4. Coat them well.
5. Place pecans on a plate lined with parchment paper. Refrigerate for 1-2 hours.
6. Serve and enjoy!

Chocolate Cake

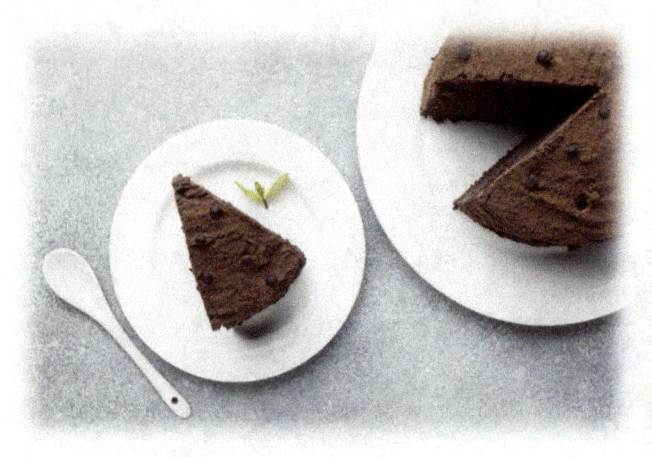

Time required: 30 minutes

Servings: 04

INGREDIENTS

1/3 cup water
3 eggs
1/3 cup sweetener, granulated
1 ½ cup almond flour, finely grated
2 tbsp cocoa powder
1 ½ tsp vanilla extract
¼ cup cocoa powder
2 ¼ tsp baking powder
A pinch of salt

STEPS FOR COOKING

1. Preheat your oven to 350F and prepare the baking sheet with parchment paper.
2. Add all the ingredients to a medium mixing bowl and stir until well combined.
3. Spread into the baking pan. Bake for approx. 10-15 minutes. Let cool before serving.
4. Enjoy!

Vanilla Pears

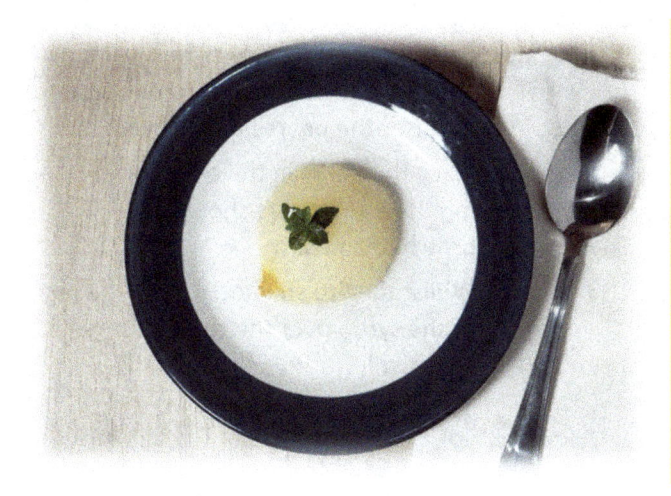

Time required: 45 minutes

Servings: 04

INGREDIENTS

4 large pears
120ml maple syrup
0.25 tsp cinnamon
1 tsp vanilla extract

STEPS FOR COOKING

1. Preheat your oven to 190 C.
2. Take a baking sheet and line it with baking parchment.
3. Take the pears and cut them into halves. Cut a small amount of the underside away, so they stand up on the baking tray.
4. Use a teaspoon to scoop out the middle of the pears and remove the seeds.
5. Arrange the pears on the baking sheet, with the middles facing upwards.
6. Sprinkle the cinnamon over the top of each pear.
7. Take a small bowl and combine the vanilla and maple syrup.

INGREDIENTS	STEPS FOR COOKING
	8. Drizzle the mixture over the pears, keeping a small amount to one side for after the pears have cooked. 9. Place the pears in the oven for 25 minutes. The pears should be browned and soft. 10. Whilst they're still hot, drizzle the rest of the syrup over the top and serve whilst still warm.

Apple Pie

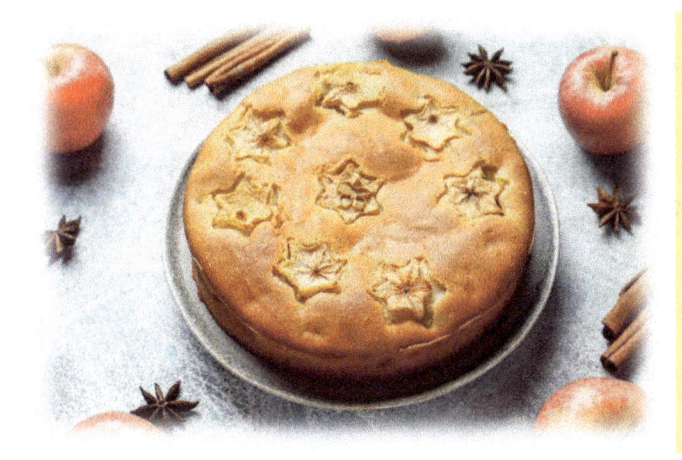

Time required: 45 minutes

Servings: 12

INGREDIENTS

For the Filling:

1 cup sweetener, granulated

1 ½ tbsp coconut flour

1 tsp cinnamon powder

4 apples, chopped

2 tbsp melted butter

1 tbsp lemon juice

1 tsp apple extract

1 9-inch keto pie crust

For the Crumble:

½ cup coconut, unsweetened, shredded

STEPS FOR COOKING

1. Preheat your oven at 350°F.
2. Prepare a pie crust.
3. In a mixing bowl add all the filling ingredients and stir until well combined.
4. Pour over the keto pie crust. Bake for approx. 20-25 minutes.
5. In a small bowl, combine all the crumble ingredients and stir well.
6. Top the cake with the crumble and bake again for approx. 10-15 minutes. Serve and enjoy!

INGREDIENTS

¼ cup brown sweetener
½ cup almonds, finely shredded
1 cup almond flour
½ cup melted coconut oil

STEPS FOR COOKING

Pumpkin Pie Flan

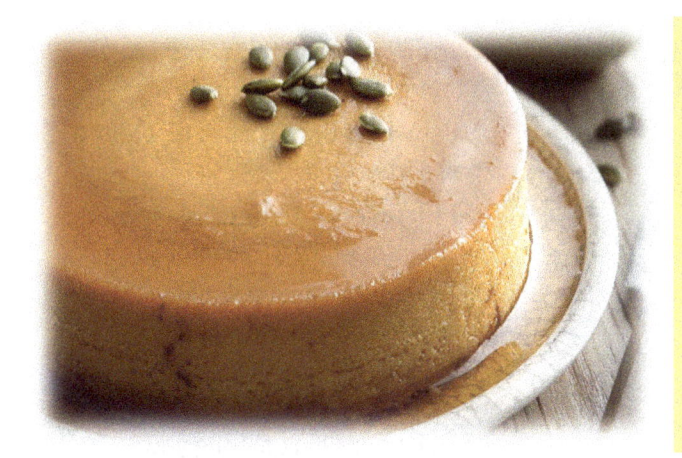

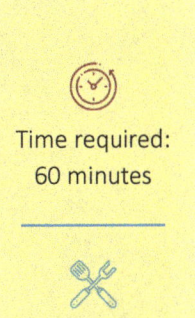

Time required: 60 minutes

Servings: 08

INGREDIENTS

2 Large Eggs
1/2 cup of Whole Milk
2 Large Egg Yolks
3/4 cup of Canned Solid-Pack Pumpkin
2/3 cup of Granulated Sugar
1 teaspoon of Vanilla Extract
1 teaspoon of Ground Cinnamon
1/4 cup of Evaporated Milk
1/2 teaspoon of Ground Nutmeg
Cooking Spray

STEPS FOR COOKING

1. Heat your oven to 350 degrees. Arrange eight 4-ounce ramekins in your 9 x 13-inch baking pan.
2. Coat your ramekins lightly with cooking spray.
3. In your small-sized saucepan, heat 1/3 cup of your sugar over medium heat, stirring constantly, until it has melted and formed a medium-brown caramel. Should take approximately 7 minutes.
4. Transfer 2 teaspoons of the caramel to each of your ramekins, swirling as soon as you spoon in your caramel. Set to the side.
5. Combine your whole milk and evaporated milk in your medium-sized saucepan over medium heat until

INGREDIENTS	STEPS FOR COOKING
	warm. Reduce your heat to a low simmer and keep warm. 6. Meanwhile, bring 4 cups of water to a boil and keep it hot. 7. Whisk together your whole eggs, egg yolks, remaining 1/3 cup of sugar, vanilla, nutmeg, and cinnamon in your medium-sized bowl. Fold in your pumpkin, then fold your pumpkin mixture into your warm milk mixture. 8. Divide your filling among your ramekins, then place your baking pan in your oven. Pour your hot water into your baking pan until it reaches halfway up the sides of your ramekins. Bake until your flan is all set. Should take approximately 35 to 40 minutes. Allow cooling completely. 9. Place your dessert plate on top of each of your ramekins and invert. 10. Serve!

Cheesecake Cupcakes

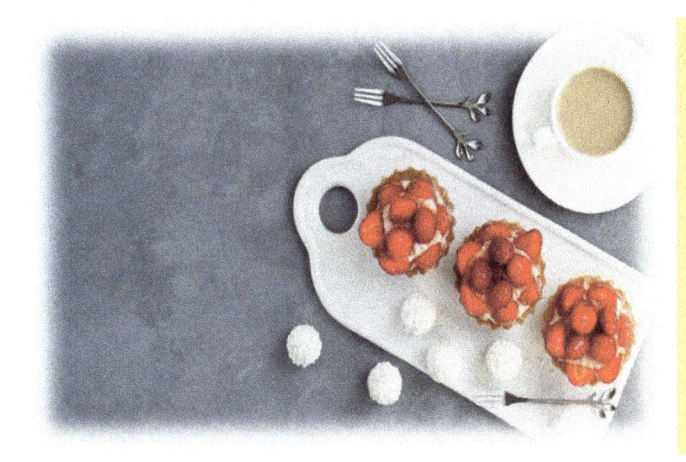

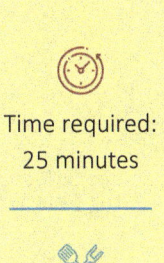

Time required: 25 minutes

Servings: 18

INGREDIENTS

For the Crust:
1 ½ cup shortbread cookies, shredded
¼ cup melted butter

For the Filling:
1 cup sour cream
2 eggs
1 tsp lemon juice
2 cups softened cream cheese
1 cup sweetener, granulated

STEPS FOR COOKING

1. Preheat your oven to 350°F and prepare 18 muffin liners in the baking dish. In a small mixing bowl combine all the crust ingredients and mix well.
2. Pour over the muffin liners. Bake for 8-10 minutes.
3. Remove from oven and reduce the heat to 300°F.
4. Beat the cream cheese in a small mixing bowl and combine with the other filling ingredients.
5. Pour the cream over the muffins. Bake for 20-25 minutes.
6. Let them cool. Serve and enjoy!

CPSIA information can be obtained
at www.ICGtesting.com
Printed in the USA
BVHW091723310521
608479BV00009B/1680

9 781802 610888